—— Second Edition ——

CODING AND PHYSICIAN LANGUAGE

Strategies for Obtaining Complete Documentation

Gloryanne Bryant, RHIA, CCS, CCDS

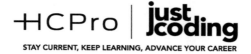

STAY CURRENT, KEEP LEARNING, ADVANCE YOUR CAREER

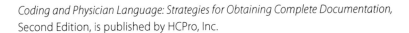

Coding and Physician Language: Strategies for Obtaining Complete Documentation, Second Edition, is published by HCPro, Inc.

ISBN: 978-1-60146-858-1

HCPro, Inc., provides information resources for the healthcare industry.

HCPro, Inc., is not affiliated in any way with The Joint Commission, which owns the JCAHO and Joint Commission trademarks.

Gloryanne Bryant, RHIA,
  CCS, CCDS, Author
Janet L. Morris, Senior Managing Editor
Ilene MacDonald, Executive Editor
Lauren McLeod, Group Publisher

Adam Carroll, Proofreader
Mike Mirabello, Senior Graphic Artist
Matt Sharpe, Production Manager
Shane Katz, Art Director
Jean St. Pierre, Senior Director of Operations

Advice given is general. Readers should consult professional counsel for specific legal, ethical, or clinical questions.

Arrangements can be made for quantity discounts. For more information, contact:

HCPro, Inc.
75 Sylvan Street, Suite A-101
Danvers, MA 01923
Telephone: 800/650-6787 or 781/639-1872
Fax: 800/639-8511
E-mail: *customerservice@hcpro.com*

To order more copies of this handbook, visit HCPro online at
***www.hcmarketplace.com* or call customer service at 800/650-6787.**

08/2011
21902

Contents

About the Author

Gloryanne Bryant, RHIA, CCS, CCDS

Bryant is a Registered Health Information Administrator (RHIA), a Registered Health Information Technician (RHIT), a Certified Coding Specialist (CCS), and a Certified Clinical Documentation Specialist (CCDS), with more than 30 years of experience in the health information management (HIM) profession. She currently is the regional managing director of HIM for the Northern California Revenue Cycle of Kaiser Permanente located in Oakland, CA. In this role, she is responsible for HIM operations, coding, coding education, and auditing, and is an advisor to clinical documentation improvement for 21 acute care facilities.

Bryant has conducted numerous workshops for hospital-based coders, covering International Classification of Diseases, 9th Revision, Clinical Modification (ICD-9-CM) and current procedural terminology (CPT) coding; diagnosis-related groups (DRG); and ambulatory payment classification (APC) (outpatient prospective payment system [OPPS]). In addition, she has made an array of presentations on data quality, medical necessity, compliance, and documentation improvement to management executives and healthcare administrators. Over the past three and a half years, she has been a guest speaker on compliance issues for several regional, state, and national educational programs and associations. She has given presentations on planning and implementation of ICD-10 during the past four years and provided testimony in support of ICD-10 implementation for the House Ways and Means Committee in April 2006.

She serves as a volunteer leader on many levels, including for the California Health Information Association (CHIA) as a director and president-elect to the state board, and has served in several national positions for the American Health Information Management Association (AHIMA). As an HIM practitioner in the HIM/coding arena, she was on the American Hospital Association Editorial Advisory Board on ICD-9-CM for *Coding Clinic* for two years.

Bryant received the CHIA Literary Award for her many articles and writings related to clinical documentation improvement, compliance, data quality, and coding. In August 2005, Bryant was appointed to the Centers for Medicare & Medicaid Services APC Advisory Panel to work on OPPS policy, coding, and reimbursement issues, where she served until August 2009. She was also appointed to the RAND Expert Panel on Severity DRGs from 2006 to 2007. She received the AHIMA Triumph Award in the category of HIM Champion in the fall of 2007.

Bryant is a sought-after national speaker and author on healthcare compliance, reimbursement, clinical documentation improvement, and coding regulations (ICD-9-CM, ICD-10, and CPT). She serves as a catalyst for change and improvement in HIM and healthcare.

Coding and Physician Language: Strategies for Obtaining Complete Documentation, Second Edition

Introduction

Clinical documentation for coding purposes continues to be highly important as we work to obtain data for quality measures and payment. Such data rely on accurate coding, which relies on complete and accurate clinical documentation; they are dependent on each other. Indeed, the more specific the documentation, the more specific the ICD-9-CM code(s) will be, and in turn, the more accurate the severity, acuity, and risk of mortality (ROM) data will be.

Clinical coding allows for the reporting of mortality data to the World Health Organization, the reporting of morbidity data in the United States, and the provision of data to third-party payers so they can reimburse hospitals for care and services provided. Coded information is also the primary source for the administrative management of medical services and a source of epidemiologic research and statistical data from inpatient stays. The National Center for Health Statistics and the Centers for Medicare & Medicaid Services (CMS) are the U.S. governmental agencies responsible for overseeing all changes and modifications to ICD-9-CM.

To ensure accurate coding, professional coders should obtain and maintain certain competencies, such as those on the American Health Information Management Association (AHIMA) list of ICD-9-CM and current procedural terminology/Healthcare Common Procedure Coding System procedural coding competencies. A sample of these competencies is listed here and at the back of this book (for a complete list, visit *www.ahima.org*):

- Knowledge of anatomy and physiology, clinical disease processes, pharmacology, and diagnostic and procedural terminology to assign accurate codes to diagnoses and procedures to reflect the services rendered

- Knowledge of disease processes and surgical procedures to assign non-indexed medical terms to the appropriate class in the classification/nomenclature system

- Knowledge of current approved ICD-9-CM coding guidelines to assign and sequence the correct diagnosis and procedure codes for hospital inpatient services

One area that coding professionals must thoroughly understand and apply is the Uniform Hospital Discharge Data Set (UHDDS) guidelines, which describe the requirement for reporting of secondary conditions or "other diagnoses" as follows:

- Clinical evaluation

- Therapeutic treatment

- Diagnostic procedures

- Extended length of hospital stay

- Increased nursing care/monitoring

Note that the coding of "chronic conditions" (including but not limited to hypertension, congestive heart failure [CHF], asthma, emphysema, chronic obstructive pulmonary disease [COPD], Parkinson's disease, and diabetes mellitus) helps capture severity of illness (SOI) and ROM. Again, reporting of chronic conditions is *not* limited to those listed here or in the American Hospital Association's (AHA) *Coding Clinic for ICD-9-CM*. Clinical documentation identifies the medical signs/ symptoms and diagnoses that are present, and for which the patient seeks or requires care and treatment.

Communication with the physician community is critical to the success of clinical documentation improvement and the capture of coded data. Although physicians take a variety of courses including pathology, physiology, and disease manifestations as part of their medical education, they are not taught the importance of "document- ing" medical terminology using details and specifics that correspond to ICD-9-CM codes. Physician profiles and scorecards are linked to ICD-9-CM codes, and the physician needs to be aware of this. To share information, there must be open lines of communication between health information management (HIM) coding professionals and the medical staff. HIM coding professionals need to be willing and able to initiate this communication and establish collaboration.

Communication between physicians and hospital HIM staff, the medical record department, and those who code in other settings (e.g., physician office, skilled nursing facility, rehabilitation) is vital as well because coding staff members must be able to query the physician when clinical documentation is not specific or needs clarification. AHIMA has developed two practice briefs related to the topic of physician queries, "Developing a Physician Query Process" and "Managing an Effective Query Process," which readers should review and keep handy as a resource. In addition, for the clinical documentation improvement arena, AHIMA published the "Clinical Documentation Improvement Program—A Model Guidance" practice brief in 2010, which serves as an excellent resource and foundational document.

Remember to code all documented conditions established upon admission and throughout the hospitalization and hospital encounter. Follow your UHDDS reporting guidelines, ICD-9-CM chapter-specific guidelines, and the ICD-9-CM coding conventions for secondary conditions. Use *AHA Coding Clinic for ICD-9-CM* for additional guidance.

Understanding the definition of "principal diagnosis" for inpatient coding is pivotal to success and data accuracy. The UHDDS defines the principal diagnosis as "that condition established after study to be chiefly responsible for occasioning the admission of the patient to the hospital for care."

Severity and risk of mortality

Clinical data is used for many purposes, but it is clear that the capture of ICD-9-CM codes has an impact on the determination of a patient's SOI and ROM. Publicly reported outcomes and projected ROM is based on clinical data that is available or purchased from state and federal agencies. Having a good understanding of SOI and ROM is important to the coding process and for quality data.

ICD-10

The transition to ICD-10-CM/PCS (procedural coding system), both diagnosis and procedure coding, is a bigger change in the U.S. healthcare system than most of us can remember. With the ICD-10 implementation date of October 1, 2013, we have lots to do to prepare. More and more organizations and vendors are developing tools and information to help increase understanding of ICD-10 implementation as well as overall awareness of the transition. Gap analysis and assessments of key work streams will be critical in the initial phase of implementation. Annual updates to ICD-9-CM will be discontinued on October 1, 2013, with limited updates in the prior year; this is done in preparation for the education being provided on the new coding system.

In preparation for ICD-10, coding professionals should determine their knowledge in the following areas:

- Medical terminology

- Anatomy and physiology

- Disease processes

- Pharmacology

These four areas have been identified as prerequisite coursework needed for successful training with ICD-10. Your ICD-10 implementation plan should include a documentation and coding assessment, a plan of action with a timeline, and several days of education and training for your coding staff. Industry experts say between 40 and 50 hours of education and training may be needed for hospital inpatient coding. Between now and October 1, 2013, there is much to be done, so having a detailed plan as well as a timeline is very important. A word of caution: Do not wait until 2013 to get ready for ICD-10!

Physician query

Coding professionals and physicians often speak two different languages, so it is critical to use a comprehensive physician query form. The documentation physicians provide often does not conform to the coding classifications system and does not always allow us to code to capture patient severity, acuity, and accurate reimbursement. Sometimes, physicians create their own terminology that is not part of the coding world or included in ICD-9-CM descriptions. In these cases, we must query the physicians for clarification.

Query forms should:

- Identify why the clarification is needed

- Present the scenario

- State the facts—just the facts

- Clarify only what is already present in the medical record

- State a question that asks the physician to make a clinical interpretation

Query forms should *NOT*:

- Be written on sticky notes or scratch paper

- Be used as a substitute for documentation in the medical record

- Lead the physician

- Ask questions that can be answered "yes" or "no"

- Indicate the financial impact

- Require only a physician signature

To ensure that medical record entries are consistent, physician queries, whether verbal or written, need to take place, but it's also important to ensure that those queries are compliant. The following areas of the medical record are important to the hospital coding process: emergency room (ER) encounter documentation (when admitted— critical for inpatient coding), history and physical (H&P), consulta- tions, assessments, treatment plans, physician progress notes, physician orders, nursing notes, medication and treatment records, admission and discharge data, pharmacy records, operative notes, and discharge summaries, just to mention a few. When one entry contradicts previous documentation, include an explanation of the contradiction in your query. Providers need to be aware of the need to adequately document the significant changes in a patient's condition or care.

Following professional ethics standards and maintaining compliance is also not to be understated. The healthcare industry is under greater scrutiny, and with the full effort of Recovery Audit Contractors (RAC) in motion, we must be especially careful and diligent.

This handbook describes important areas related to documentation and coding of common diagnoses/conditions and provides information to help in achieving a better understanding of these conditions, especially in relation to the inpatient hospital setting. However, the handbook is not all-inclusive. Therefore, remember that accurate coding can be achieved only with specific and detailed clinical documentation coupled with educated and trained coding staff. The coding golden rule and compliance standard is, "If it isn't documented, you can't code it."

Acute Myocardial Infarction

- Review the medical record documentation carefully for specific signs and symptoms relating to a myocardial infarction (MI) (e.g., elevated troponin [cardiac enzymes], electrocardiogram changes, radiating chest pain or arm pain) when the patient presents with chest pain.

- Look in the 410.0x–410.6x series for the ICD-9-CM codes for a transmural (full thickness) acute MI. ICD-9-CM provides a wide range of codes to choose from, so check the documentation carefully. The code 410.7x identifies the infarction as subendocardial, which means that it did not extend to the full thickness of the myocardial wall.

- Use code 410.9 to describe an MI for which the site is "unspecified." Do not assign this code unless there is no further clarifying documentation in the medical record or from a physician query. However, the fifth-digit subclassification is still needed.

- Use the fifth-digit subclassification for 410.xx, which reflects the episode of care (e.g., current, subsequent, or unspecified). Assign the fifth digit "0" for unspecified episode of care only when the documentation fails to provide further information or specifics.

- Review the clinical documentation carefully when an MI evolves into right ventricular failure and progresses to CHF.

- Review nursing notes, especially those from the intensive care or cardiac care unit. This information often indicates other conditions that the patient is being treated for but that the physician did not document because the condition resolved by the time he or she saw the patient again. Audits indicate that arrhythmias (e.g., atrial fibrillation) often occur but are not coded due to the lack of physician documentation; however, using a query may help clarify the condition that nursing staff may be treating.

- Watch the documentation for "postmyocardial infarction hypotension" (code 458.8, other specified hypotension).

- Be sure to review the documentation for the time frame of when the acute MI occurred as this can impact the code selection.

- Acute MI is one of the "core measures" quality diagnoses; thus, care should be taken when selecting acute MI as the principal diagnosis.

- Look for MI codes in Chapter 7, "Diseases of Circulatory System (390–459)," in ICD-9-CM, Sixth Edition, valid from October 1, 2010, to September 30, 2011.

Adverse Effects of Medications

- Sometimes the terminology used by a physician does not correlate to the terms used by ICD-9-CM (e.g., toxicity vs. poisoning vs. adverse effect). Understand the coding guidelines regarding adverse effects and follow the indexing properly.

- Review the clinical documentation carefully when a condition is due to a drug, medicinal, or biological substance (e.g., an allergic reaction due to a drug or an arrhythmia due to a prescribed medication).

- Code the adverse effect first when the correct substance was administered as prescribed but it resulted in an adverse effect, which is often a sign or symptom.

- Use the ICD-9-CM 960–979 code series when a substance was used incorrectly and the case is classified as a poisoning (poisoning by drugs, medicinal and biological substances).

- Review the medical record documentation for any drug interactions that may have occurred.

- Always code the drug(s) responsible for an adverse effect (codes E930–E949) when documented.

- Review the documentation in the medical record carefully or query the physician for further clarification when he or she uses the term "toxic effect" or "toxicity," which often means that there is an adverse effect caused by a correctly administered, prescribed drug.

Alcohol/Substance Use/Abuse

- Often, the medical record H&P will mention or describe the patient's social history, which may include the use of alcohol. This is an area of documentation that should be reviewed closely and carefully.

- Seek clarification (query) from the physician, if necessary, when the medical record indicates that the patient sometimes drinks alcohol but does not have a problem, or does not state whether there is any abuse or dependence.

- Seek more specific documentation when coding an alcohol abuse or dependence ICD-9-CM code if the documentation indicates periodic or episodic abuse (e.g., weekend drinker) or if the patient is alcohol-dependent. The diagnosis of "alcoholism," unspecified, codes to 303.9, other and unspecified alcohol dependence, with a fifth-digit subclassification to indicate the type of abuse. However, the fifth-digit subclassification is still needed.

- Ask the physician to specify or document whether the patient has other body system effects of alcohol or drug abuse or dependence, and name the related disease process.

- Clarify with the physician whether the patient is an occasional abuser or is dependent on alcohol or drugs.

- Educate physicians that documenting or writing "+ coc", "+ barb", and/or "– ETOH" does not provide enough information for coding. Coding staff may not apply codes from a positive laboratory test, per coding guidelines. Physicians should document whether the patient suffers from substance abuse and, if so, name the substance.

- Assign the following ICD-9-CM procedure codes to the medical record when there is documentation of therapy for alcohol abuse and dependence:

  - 94.61, alcohol rehabilitation

- 94.62, alcohol detoxification

- 94.63, alcohol rehabilitation and detoxification

- Assign the following ICD-9-CM procedure codes when there is documentation of therapy for drug abuse and dependence:

  - 94.64, drug rehabilitation

  - 94.65, drug detoxification

  - 94.66, drug rehabilitation and detoxification

- Assign the following ICD-9-CM combined therapy codes when indicated if patients have both alcohol and drug usage and therapy:

  - 94.67, combined alcohol and drug rehabilitation

  - 94.68, combined alcohol and drug detoxification

  - 94.69, combined alcohol and drug rehabilitation and detoxification

- Look for ICD-9-CM codes relating to alcohol or drug abuse treatment in Chapter 5, "Mental Disorders (290–319)," and in the procedure chapter, "Miscellaneous Diagnostic and Therapeutic Procedures (87–99)," in ICD-9-CM, Sixth Edition, valid from October 1, 2010, to September 30, 2011.

Anemia

- The coding of anemia has been a long-standing challenge for hospital coding professionals. Obtaining specificity is also a challenge with capturing the appropriate ICD-9-CM code(s) for anemia. Although findings from a laboratory study may indicate an abnormal range of hemoglobin (hgb) or hematocrit (hct), the physician needs to provide an interpretation or document the significance of that abnormal finding. A coding professional cannot assume or make a diagnosis.

- Watch for the term "anemia" in the ER documentation and H&P. Although it's not specific, finding the term "anemia" is one of the first steps to take when coding. Then review the clinical documentation carefully, including the progress notes and physician orders.

- It can be useful to review the laboratory findings, particularly the hgb/hct. Review the physician's orders for testing/monitoring or for procedures related to the condition of anemia.

- Review the blood values following a surgical procedure when coding a medical record in which surgery was performed. Look at the hgb/hct to see whether it has dropped significantly and whether monitoring is occurring. In the absence of documentation for anemia or acute blood loss anemia, query the physician for a specific diagnosis relating to this finding. Remember, coding guidelines prohibit coders from coding from laboratory findings and values alone.

- Clarify, if necessary, the underlying cause of the anemia (e.g., due to long-term anticoagulants, gastric ulcer, neoplasm, or internal bleeding), as it will make a difference in the ICD-9-CM code that is assigned.*

- Look for anemia codes in Chapter 4, "Diseases of Blood and Blood-Forming Organs (280–289)," in ICD-9-CM, Sixth Edition, valid from October 1, 2010, to September 30, 2011.

Review and follow AHA Coding Clinic for ICD-9-CM *guidance and information relating to the coding of anemia and specific types of anemia.*

Body Mass Index

- The ICD-9-CM official coding guidelines discuss the coding of body mass index (BMI). In addition, *AHA Coding Clinic for ICD-9-CM* has discussed the coding of BMI, so this guidance should also be reviewed and followed.

- Coders should not calculate the BMI.

- Base the BMI code assignment on medical record documentation, which may be found in the physician documentation, dietitian's notes, or other nonphysician provider notes. Note that this is an exception to the coding guideline that requires coders to base code assignment on the documentation by the physician or any qualified healthcare practitioner who is legally accountable for establishing the patient's diagnosis.

- Although coders may report BMI based on the dietitian's or other caregiver's documentation, coders must base the diagnosis codes for overweight and obesity on the physician's documentation.

- You should not code the BMI without a related diagnosis/ condition code.

- BMI is in the V85 subcategory. These V codes are used to capture the BMI for adults over 20 years old and for pediatric patients 2–20 years of age.

Chest Pain/Angina

- Educate coders about the implications of chest pain, which is a common chief complaint in the ER.

- Documentation needs to be specific so the chest pain can be coded to the most specific code possible. There are several different classifications of chest pain in ICD-9-CM (e.g., musculoskeletal, respiratory, precordial).

- Documentation should indicate the underlying cause of the chest pain when known. Specific types of chest pain (e.g., cardiac or noncardiac) must be supported by the physician documentation. Query the physician for the underlying cause of the chest pain.

- Be aware that the presenting symptom of chest pain is often diagnosed as angina, which is a manifestation of ischemic heart disease or an MI.

- If the physician diagnoses angina, query for further clarification as to the cause of the angina (e.g., coronary artery disease [CAD]).

- Review the documentation for a specific type of angina because there are several classifications of angina with different ICD-9-CM codes.

- Query the physician for a more specific type of angina if the principal diagnosis in the inpatient record simply states "angina." Documentation of a more specific type of angina (e.g., unstable, stable, Prinzmetal) can affect the code assignment, severity, and acuity/severity of the case.

- Look for angina codes in Chapter 7, "Diseases of Circulatory System (390–459)," in ICD-9-CM, Sixth Edition, valid from October 1, 2010, to September 30, 2011.

Chronic Obstructive Pulmonary Disease

- Be aware that chronic obstructive pulmonary disease (COPD) is a progressive disease that can exacerbate to an acute condition, which may ultimately result in oxygen dependence and in end-stage disease. Documentation should reflect the stage of the lung disease for accurate coding.

- Assign code 496, chronic airway obstruction, not elsewhere classified, even when there is only documentation to support this code in the history of the patient, per guidelines found in *AHA Coding Clinic for ICD-9-CM*. Because COPD is a chronic condition that affects the patient for the rest of his or her life, report and code it when documented in the medical record. Do the same for other chronic conditions, such as diabetes mellitus, hypertension, and Parkinson's disease.

- Assign the appropriate ICD-9-CM code for COPD when the anesthesiologist documents it. *AHA Coding Clinic for ICD-9-CM* instructs the coder that "coding is based on physician documentation; the anesthesiologist is a physician. However, if there is conflicting information in the record, query the attending physician for clarification."

- Review the documentation to see whether historical information reveals that the patient has acute bronchitis versus acute exacerbation of chronic bronchitis, stable COPD, or other chronic lung disease.

- Assign code 496, chronic airway obstruction, not elsewhere classified, to describe chronic obstructive lung disease, a condition in which there is chronic obstruction to airflow due to chronic bronchitis/emphysema. This code excludes chronic obstructive lung disease or COPD specified as obstructive chronic bronchitis, chronic asthmatic bronchitis, asthma with chronic obstruction, and emphysema.

- Review the clinical documentation carefully as there are situations in which a patient with COPD also will have acute respiratory failure upon admission, even though he or she may not have required intubation or mechanical ventilation.

- Be sure to note what the respiratory treatment consists of. If, for example, the patient is receiving bi-level positive airway pressure (BiPAP), this may be an indication of a worsening respiratory condition.

- Look for COPD codes in Chapter 8, "Diseases of Respiratory System (460–519)," in ICD-9-CM, Sixth Edition, valid from October 1, 2010, to September 30, 2011.

Comfort Care or Palliative Care

- Comfort care, end-of-life care, and palliative care are presented in ICD-9-CM using code V66.7. *AHA Coding Clinic for ICD-9-CM* has published instructions and information relating to comfort/palliative care.

- Please refer to *Coding Clinic,* First Quarter 1998, pp. 11–12, Effective with Discharges: January 15, 1998, and *Coding Clinic,* Third Quarter 2008, pp. 13–14, Effective with Discharges: September 19, 2008, as resources.

- Palliative care is extended to terminally ill patients, such as those with cancer. However, a terminal illness can also be a condition such as end-stage COPD or end-stage CHF. Palliative care rendered at earlier times within a terminal illness disease process can be coded regardless of when it is ordered within a patient's care continuum.

- When the palliative care team orders and treats a patient for palliative care, assign the code V66.7 for palliative care as a secondary diagnosis. The terminal condition should be the principal or secondary diagnosis depending on the admission and circumstances.

- The V66.7 code is often used when determining the ROM, so V66.7 needs to be in the top 25 diagnosis codes in order to be captured via Medicare Provider Analysis and Review (MedPAR) data and for other analysis.

Comorbidities

- Understand the definition of comorbidity, meaning a preexisting condition. These conditions can also be referred to as "chronic systemic conditions."

- Report comorbid diagnoses as secondary conditions/diagnoses to help capture severity, acuity, and ROM in addition to the impact on case-mix index and payment.

- Review the documentation in the H&P or consultation report for information about other diseases the patient may have that the attending physician or another physician is following, and code those diseases/conditions. Refer to specific coding guidelines in *AHA Coding Clinic for ICD-9-CM*.

- Review the clinical documentation related to the evaluation, treatment (i.e., medications ordered), and required ongoing monitoring of conditions; code and report this information. If the documentation does not reflect the condition being treated, query the physician for clarification. Remember, however, that you can code a diagnosis from the physician order per *AHA Coding Clinic for ICD-9-CM*.

- Code all documented conditions (e.g., risk factors) that could affect the patient's ability to tolerate surgery, could result in problems during or after an operation, or could affect the hospitalization.

Coronary Artery Disease

- Assign code 414.01, coronary atherosclerosis, of native coronary artery, if medical record documentation shows no history of prior coronary artery bypass. If the documentation is unclear concerning prior bypass surgery, *AHA Coding Clinic for ICD-9-CM*, Second Quarter 1995, advises coders to query the physician.

- Review the documentation to determine whether the patient has coronary occlusive disease. The physician should specify whether it is the cause of cardiomyopathy or chest pain, if present. You may need to query him or her.

- Query the physician, if necessary, if the patient has had a coronary artery bypass graft and is symptomatic but the physician does not specify whether the symptoms are due to disease of the remaining native vessels or occlusion of bypass vein, artery, or other graft. Name the vessel or graft material, if known.

- Use code 411.1 when a patient has acute coronary syndrome (ACS). This condition includes unstable angina (code 411.1) and requires immediate medical treatment. Sometimes physicians will use the terms CAD and acute coronary syndrome interchangeably.

- Find codes for CAD in Chapter 7, "Diseases of Circulatory System (390–459)," in ICD-9-CM, Sixth Edition, valid from October 1, 2010, to September 30, 2011.

Debridement

- Be aware that within ICD-9-CM procedure coding, there are two main codes for debridement (86.22, excisional debridement, and 86.28, nonexcisional debridement) of burn, infection, or wound, but only excisional debridement (86.22) can significantly affect severity acuity data and change the Medicare severity diagnosis-related group (MS-DRG). Nonexcisional debridement is the removal of devitalized tissue via washing, brushing, or flushing, while excisional debridement is the removal of devitalized tissue using a sharp instrument (e.g., scissors, scalpel, or similar tool/technique).

- Procedure code 86.22 has been a target for RACs due to the high MS-DRG reimbursement that can result from this code and the ongoing documentation issues that have been identified.

- Review all clinical documentation carefully and maintain open lines of communication with physicians and nonphysician clinicians (e.g., nurses, physical therapists, wound care staff) because the ICD-9-CM coding guidelines allow for the coding of excisional debridement when performed by both physicians and nonphysician clinicians. You may want to reach out to your nonphysician providers of wound care services and discuss the documentation issues.

- Review the clinical documentation and note where the services are being provided. Watch for a diagnosis of "ulcer," "wound," or "infected wound." Use the code for excisional debridement (86.22) if the procedure was performed with scissors or a scalpel/curette with a goal of removing necrotic or devitalized tissue from a wound (such as an ulcer), infection, or burn.

- Do not code "debridement" if a procedure merely involves cleaning up the edges of a laceration prior to closure.

- Review the documentation to determine the specifics of the procedure (e.g., debridement of toenails versus debridement of a foot ulcer).

- Review the changes in the MS-DRGs for fiscal year 2012 regarding the operative impact of ICD-9-CM code 86.22.

Delirium With Dementia

- There are several types of delirium within ICD-9-CM, including acute delirium, alcohol delirium, drug-induced delirium, transient delirium, and uremic delirium.

- Note that "delirium" and "acute confusional state" are often considered interchangeable terms.

- Delirium can be associated with other diseases and conditions (e.g., Alzheimer's disease, alcoholism, drug use, senility, and arteriosclerosis).

- Query the physician for clarification if the documentation does not clearly specify the type of delirium or the associated disease and/or condition.

Dementia

- Be aware that dementia is characterized by the development of multiple cognitive deficits, such as memory impairment or functional impairment, and cognitive disturbances, such as aphasia, apraxia, or agnosis. Examine the daily progress notes documentation and the review of systems closely.

- Understand that dementia is often a symptom of something else, such as generalized cerebrovascular ischemia, Alzheimer's disease, or toxic effects of drugs. Coders may need to ask the physician to identify the likely cause of the patient's presentation and query regarding the treatment or care of that cause. The documentation should clearly identify the relationship in the medical record.

- When querying the physician, ask for the specific reason or cause relationship of the dementia. There may be times when the dementia is related to an infection, sepsis, dehydration, or specific organ failure. If necessary, query the physician to obtain clarifying documentation that addresses the specific reason for cause relationship between a condition and the mental status change.

- Coding guidelines state that when assigning codes 294.10 and 294.11, the underlying disease associated with the dementia (such as Alzheimer's disease or Huntington's disease) should be coded first.

- Because advances in the treatment and study of dementia have allowed for the expansion of dementia code classifications, ICD-9-CM contains codes for several different types of dementia. Report separately any behavioral disturbance associated with these dementias using the appropriate code (294.10–294.11).

Fracture Reduction of Femur

- Review the documentation in the operative note carefully to properly code a surgical reduction of a femur fracture. Do not assign a code simply from the title of the procedure or operation. Pay attention to the operative details and the narrative portion of the operative report, and note whether there was a reduction prior to the incision being made.

- Make sure the clinical documentation defines when the fracture was reduced because ICD-9-CM procedure codes for inpatient coding require specific information. Sometimes, surgeons will use the language of a closed reduction when they actually mean an open reduction with internal fixation; this inaccuracy could result in an incorrect code assignment.

- Be aware that although patients may lose blood at the fracture site, findings of a significant drop in hgb/hct is not a complication of the surgery. However, if the patient loses enough blood from the fracture site to warrant monitoring, follow-up, or transfusion, look for documentation of a diagnosis, such as anemia or other clinical indications of a condition, or consider querying the physician for the diagnostic condition that warrants the monitoring, follow-up, or transfusion. Keep in mind that blood loss relating to the fracture site is an acute post-traumatic hemorrhagic anemia.

- You may need to query the physician if the surgeon does not document other chronic, stable conditions that are under treatment but are being followed by another physician while the patient is in the hospital.

For example, conditions such as acute urinary retention, atelectasis, or volume overload may be present with clinical findings but not documented as a condition or diagnosis. Coding guidelines state that coding from a consultant's note is acceptable as long as there is no conflicting diagnostic information from the primary physician.

Gastrointestinal Bleed

- Query the physician if he or she documents "gastrointestinal [GI] bleed," as you may need to know whether the GI bleed is causing anemia. If there is documentation of "anemia," you may need to request supporting documentation as to whether the diagnosis is acute blood loss anemia, chronic blood loss anemia, or another specific type.

- Ask the physician to provide documentation as to the cause of the bleed and whether it is upper or lower GI. Sometimes the physician does not know which one it is until he or she conducts studies (i.e., an endoscopy or colonoscopy). If an endoscopy or colonoscopy was performed in the presence of a GI bleed, you will need to review the procedure documentation carefully, as there may be an indication in the findings from that report. Remember, rectal bleeds originate in the rectum. If the physician uses the terms "melena" or "hematochezia," think of the rectal region in relation to the site and proper code assignment. Seek clarification from the physician if in doubt.

- Follow the ICD-9-CM guidelines for coding GI hemorrhage, which can manifest itself in several ways:

  - Hematemesis, indicating acute upper GI hemorrhage

  - Melena, indicating upper or lower GI hemorrhage

- Occult, bleeding seen on laboratory examination only

- Hematochezia, usually indicating blood in the rectum

- Be aware that when a patient presents with acute hemorrhage (which can manifest as significant hematemesis, melena, or hematochezia), the initial focus of treatment is usually an assessment and restoration of the individual's blood volume using IV fluids and blood transfusions as needed. This also could indicate that a possible condition of anemia is present, warranting a query.

- When coding a medical record in which the patient presents with GI hemorrhage due to an identified cause, the code sequencing depends on the circumstances of admission. If the thrust of treatment—based on the documentation, including diagnostic procedures—is directed toward control of the bleeding, identify the GI hemorrhage as the principal or primary diagnosis. Carefully review the circumstances of the encounter or admission to help with determining the appropriate diagnosis code.

- However, if the bleeding is minimal and easily controlled, and the documentation indicates that the major thrust of treatment is directed toward the underlying cause, code and list that underlying condition as principal/primary diagnosis with an additional code for the bleed. In some situations, one ICD-9-CM code includes both the identified cause and the hemorrhage. Refer to specific coding guidelines in *AHA Coding Clinic for ICD-9-CM*.

Heart Failure

- There is a greater emphasis and scrutiny on patients with CHF due to core measures, readmission rates, and other quality initiatives. Accurate documentation and coding is vital for these efforts and for data integrity.

- Understand the clinical aspects of heart failure to assign the correct ICD-9-CM code. Heart failure occurs when the heart is unable to pump sufficient blood throughout the body. Some of the common and frequently documented signs and symptoms of heart failure are edema, fatigue, and dyspnea (shortness of breath) at rest or during exercise.

- Review the documentation for the results of cardiac function studies and determine whether, according to the physician, the reports reflect failure due to left ventricular systolic dysfunction, left ventricular diastolic dysfunction, or both. Clarify with the physician if necessary.

- Determine whether the current episode reflects acute decompensation (e.g., a patient with chronic diastolic failure due to hypertensive heart disease with acute systolic decompensation due to subendocardial MI).

- Be aware that in October 2002, ICD-9-CM code category 428, heart failure, was modified to provide greater specificity regarding the type of heart failure (e.g., congestive, systolic, diastolic, and combined diastolic and systolic). Also, several subcategories were further divided to identify whether the heart failure is unspecified, acute, chronic, or acute on chronic (which refers to a patient who has CHF and also experiences an acute flare-up).

- Query the physician, if necessary, to document whether the heart failure is systolic or diastolic. Because there are different long-term treatments, differentiating between systolic and diastolic dysfunction better captures severity and acuity.

- CHF is one of the "core measures" quality diagnoses; thus, care should be taken when selecting CHF as the principal diagnosis. Meet with your core measures staff to discuss the documentation requirements—this will help them as well.

- Find codes for heart failure in Chapter 7, "Diseases of Circulatory System (390–459)," in ICD-9-CM, Sixth Edition, valid from October 1, 2010, to September 30, 2011.

Hyperglycemia

- Review the hemoglobin A1c findings to determine what the physician documentation reflects: Does the patient have controlled or uncontrolled diabetes? If necessary, query the physician.

- Look for certain terminology. For example, type 1 diabetes refers to the body's lack of insulin production. Type 2 refers to a resistance to insulin. In the case of a patient with adult-onset diabetes taking insulin, the physician documentation should state "type 2 taking insulin" and not "insulin dependence."

Physicians should avoid stating "IDDM" (insulin-dependent diabetes mellitus) and "NIDDM" (non-insulin-dependent diabetes mellitus).

- Review the documentation carefully to determine whether the patient has other manifestations of diabetes (e.g., gastroparesis, diabetic renal failure, blindness, or neuropathy). It is fairly common for patients with diabetes to also have manifestations depending on the length of the diabetic history and the severity, but these manifestations will also need to be documented and coded.

- If the patient is not diabetic, query the physician if he or she has not documented the reason for hyperglycemia (e.g., steroid therapy, other endocrine dysfunction).

- Remember that insulin therapy may be required in some cases to correct symptomatic or persistent hyperglycemia.

- Review the documentation carefully or query the physician, if necessary, to determine whether hyperglycemia occurred in secondary diabetes induced by steroid use.

- Find codes for diabetes in Chapter 3, "Endocrine, Nutritional, and Metabolic Diseases and Immunity Disorders (240–279)," in ICD-9-CM, Sixth Edition, valid from October 1, 2010, to September 30, 2011.

Low Anterior Resection

- Look for physician documentation, which should define whether the disease process originated in the sigmoid colon, in the rectum, or at the rectosigmoid junction. This could be documentation in the operative report.

- Review the documentation for indications of diverticular disease. Look carefully for an indication that the disease may be of the sigmoid colon or rectum.

- Review whether the surgeon specified which part of the bowel was resected (e.g., sigmoidectomy, rectal resection), as this information can affect the ICD-9-CM procedure code and makes the data more valuable. Do not assign the ICD-9-CM procedure code based on the title of the operation or on the title of the operative report.

- Review the operative report for an indication of a possible colostomy with a low anterior resection.

- Review the pathology report for verification that a rectal resection was performed. In many cases, the resection is actually of the colon and not of the rectum.

Malignancies

- In reference to a malignancy, review physician documentation that states "history of," which could indicate that the malignancy is still present. The language used by physicians may not be a true representation of the state of the malignancy. Physician documentation should identify the primary source of the malignancy and whether that primary source is still being treated or has been treated and is no longer present.

- Review the physician documentation to determine whether there is a recurrence at the same site or reappearance at a different site (i.e., metastasis), and if so, where.

- Query the physician, if necessary, to determine whether current symptoms are related to direct invasion of the malignancy, related to the pressure effect, or totally unrelated to the presence of the malignancy.

- Remember that the words "mass" and "tumor" do not mean "cancer." Coders may need to clarify with the physician whether a scan or x-ray shows malignancy before documenting the malignancy in the medical record.

Malnutrition

- Review physician documentation for the presence of malnutrition when it exists in cases involving unplanned weight loss in a short span of time, and look for documentation to indicate whether it is mild, moderate, or severe (20% or more of body mass lost) malnutrition. Look for physician documentation to describe the cause of the malnutrition (e.g., due to colon cancer with widespread liver metastases).

- Nutritional deficiencies (260–269) include the degree of malnutrition: mild, moderate, severe, and unspecified.

- Read the ICD-9-CM classification of malnutrition carefully. Note that ICD-9-CM code 260, kwashiorkor or "protein malnutrition," is not a common type of malnutrition seen in the United States. This condition is a nutritional edema with dyspigmentation of the skin and hair. Review the documentation and the indexing of the term used by the physician. Query the physician if there is conflicting or contrasting documentation.

- Protein-calorie malnutrition includes a biochemical change in the electrolytes, lipids, and blood plasma, and has specific codes within ICD-9-CM.

- In patients with chronic protein losses, whether through gastrointestinal losses, renal losses, or burn cases, review physician documentation for a patient who may have protein-calorie malnutrition.

- In patients with severe trauma or infectious disease or after complex surgeries requiring prolonged time without sufficient nutritional intake, review physician documentation to indicate when acute malnutrition exists due to trauma, infection, or surgery.

- In cases of child or elder abuse or various cases of purposeful or pathologic undereating, review physician documentation to determine whether malnutrition exists and whether it is mild, moderate, or severe.

- In pediatric cases with failure to thrive for whatever reason, review documentation specifically when malnutrition exists and clarify whether it is mild, moderate, or severe malnutrition.

- Find codes for malnutrition in Chapter 3, "Endocrine, Nutritional, and Metabolic Diseases and Immunity Disorders (240–279)," in ICD-9-CM, Sixth Edition, valid from October 1, 2010, to September 30, 2011.

Obesity

- Obesity is most often classified to code 278.00 (unspecified), but there are a few other more specific codes to choose from.

- Morbid obesity is coded to ICD-9-CM 278.01.

- Documentation of "overweight" is coded to 278.02.

- Pickwickian syndrome, also called "obesity hypoventilation syndrome," is coded to 278.03.

- A diagnosis of "morbid obesity" may have a BMI documented also, so be sure to review the dietary documentation as well.

- Find codes for obesity in Chapter 3, "Endocrine, Nutritional, and Metabolic Diseases and Immunity Disorders (240–279)," in ICD-9-CM, Sixth Edition, valid from October 1, 2010, to September 30, 2011.

Pneumonia

- Be aware that pneumonia coding for the inpatient setting has been under scrutiny for more than 10 years, and the Office of Inspector General continues to investigate and scrutinize pneumonia coding due to upcoding reportedly found for pneumonia MS-DRGs. Pneumonia is a fairly common diagnosis in the hospital setting, but obtaining specificity for this diagnosis can be a challenge.

- Look at the coding guidelines published in *AHA Coding Clinic for ICD-9-CM,* Second Quarter 1998, which provide specific details regarding the proper coding of a pneumonia diagnosis. This issue provides helpful information about the documentation needed as well as the correct code assignment.

- Do not assume a certain type of pneumonia is present based on the laboratory examination or results.

- Look for the physician to link the organism or cause (e.g., *Klebsiella*) of the pneumonia before you assign the specific pneumonia type (e.g., pneumonia due to *Klebsiella,* 482.0).

- Remember that a Gram stain is not conclusive evidence of a Gram-negative pneumonia. If the physician documented that the patient has pneumonia, he or she also should document in the medical record that this pneumonia is Gram-negative before you assign the code 482.83, other Gram-negative bacteria. When no additional information is available or the physician does not reply to a query, assign code 486, pneumonia, unspecified.

- Note whether the patient was admitted from a skilled nursing facility or has a history of a cerebrovascular accident (CVA) with dysphagia, which could be indicative of an aspiration. Aspiration pneumonia often can be present without physician documentation, so a query would be necessary to obtain specific documentation.

- Assign code 486, pneumonia, unspecified, when the organism is not identified and there is no further documentation that provides specificity.

- Pneumonia is one of the "core measures" quality diagnoses; thus, care should be taken when selecting pneumonia as the principal diagnosis. Meet with your core measure staff to discuss the documentation requirement—this will help them as well.

- Look for pneumonia codes in Chapter 8, "Diseases of Respiratory System (460–519)," in ICD-9-CM, Sixth Edition, valid from October 1, 2010, to September 30, 2011.

Postoperative Complications

- Review the documentation on the operative report/note and determine whether complications occurred during the surgery and required corrective action.

- Do not assume there is a complication without supporting documentation. You may need to query the physician for clarification if the documentation is unclear or conflicting.

- Often, the physician's documentation and language is merely reflecting the time frame after the surgery by documenting "postop," so use caution when choosing a postoperative complication code.

- Review the *Coding Clinic* guidance relating to specific examples of postoperative complications.

- Avoid being dependent on encoders; review the clinical documentation and indications carefully.

- Complication codes can have an impact on quality scores; therefore, care needs to be taken before assigning an ICD-9-CM postoperative complication code.

Pulmonary Edema

- Assign postoperative pulmonary edema, not otherwise specified (without adult respiratory distress syndrome), to ICD-9-CM code 518.4, unless documentation indicates the pulmonary edema is due to left ventricular failure (428.1) or CHF (428.0).

- Code postoperative pulmonary edema due to fluid overload as 518.4 and 276.6; follow *AHA Coding Clinic for ICD-9-CM* guidelines.

- Determine whether documentation indicates that there is volume overload related to renal failure with an otherwise stable heart. If present, the physician should document it as "noncardiac pulmonary edema is present." If the documentation is unclear, query the physician.

- Remember that postoperative pulmonary edema with adult respiratory distress syndrome is assigned to 518.5.

Renal Failure

- ICD-9-CM has changed the classification of renal failure over the past several years and has designated the stage of chronic renal failure (CRF) in the classification system. Capturing the stage of renal failure can properly indicate the severity and ROM.

- Educate physicians that they must avoid using the term "renal insufficiency" if they actually mean renal failure. If the patient does have renal insufficiency, the physician should specify it as "acute" or "chronic" because renal insufficiency alone does not index in ICD-9-CM. Use the written query process, if necessary, to help obtain specific documentation relating to renal insufficiency that is acute, chronic, or due to a procedure.

- Review physician documentation in the medical record for an elevation of blood urea nitrogen and creatinine as a transient event due to mild dehydration or obstruction, and document the cause of the azotemia. Query the physician as needed for additional documentation or clarification.

- Remember that, clinically, for irreversible CRF or chronic renal disease, the treatment of choice documented in the medical record might be either dialysis or transplantation. The diagnosis of acute renal failure or acute renal disease may be temporary, and the patient's renal function may recover after certain interventions, including dialysis.

- Remember that the physician documentation should reflect the stage of chronic kidney disease in patients with chronic renal insufficiency or CRF; this will help in assigning an ICD-9-CM code that correctly reflects the severity, acuity, and ROM.

- Be sure that when a patient has hypertension and renal disease/failure, the documentation reflects whether the renal disease is from another cause. To avoid incorrect coding, query the physician for clarification if necessary.

- Find codes for renal failure in Chapter 10, "Diseases of Genitourinary System (580–629)," in ICD-9-CM, Sixth Edition, valid from October 1, 2010, to September 30, 2011.

Respiratory Failure

- Review the clinical documentation in the medical record carefully when the patient has a diagnosis of respiratory failure, in addition to any other diagnoses. Often we hear that coding audits identify that respiratory failure is missed in the coding process.

- Look for documentation to specify whether the respiratory failure is acute or chronic, or if chronic respiratory failure with acute decompensation (acute on chronic) is present. You may need to query the physician for the specific degree of respiratory failure.

- Determine whether documentation identifies the basic disease causing the respiratory failure or the acute process on top of a chronic disease (e.g., acute respiratory failure due to pneumonia in a patient with chronic respiratory failure from multiple sclerosis).

- Review the respiratory failure guidelines published in *AHA Coding Clinic for ICD-9-CM,* which provides specific coding and sequencing guidelines.

- Review the progress notes and discharge summary to determine whether the patient had acute respiratory failure upon admission.

- Know the clinical indicators for respiratory failure. Be sure to review the respiratory therapy treatment notes. BiPAP respiratory therapy treatment could be an indication of respiratory failure, and a physician query may be needed.

- Review the ICD-9-CM chapter-specific coding guidelines (e.g., obstetrics, poisoning, HIV, newborn) that provide sequencing directions that take precedence. Note that respiratory failure may be listed as a secondary diagnosis if it occurs after admission.

- Find codes for respiratory failure in Chapter 8, "Diseases of Respiratory System (460–519)," in ICD-9-CM, Sixth Edition, valid from October 1, 2010, to September 30, 2011.

Seizures

- Look to see whether the documentation states that the patient had a seizure (postictal state) or other cause of alteration of consciousness.

- Review documentation to see whether the physician indicates the relationship between other existing diseases and the seizure (e.g., recent or old stroke, recent or old head trauma, brain tumor, febrile convulsion, drug overdose, alcoholism, diabetes out of control, viral or other infection, sepsis).

- Clarify with the physician, if necessary, whether a respiratory condition prompted admission of a known seizure patient who aspirated at the time of the seizure event.

- Determine whether the physician believes that the patient has epilepsy. If he or she does, the physician should document it to differentiate from other causes of seizure. The physician should name the type (e.g., partial epilepsy, grand mal, petit mal).

- Look for the code for the diagnosis of "seizure, unspecified" (code 780.39) in Chapter 16, "Signs, Symptoms and Ill-Defined Conditions (780–799)," in ICD-9-CM, Sixth Edition, valid from October 1, 2010, to September 30, 2011.

Sepsis

- There are specific instructions in the *Official Guidelines for Coding and Reporting* on septicemia, systemic inflammatory response syndrome (SIRS), sepsis, severe sepsis, and septic shock. Coding staff need to review these guidelines carefully.

- Understand the clinical signs and symptoms of sepsis and severe sepsis. Review information provided by *AHA Coding Clinic for ICD-9-CM* on the coding of sepsis and severe sepsis.

- Understand that the definition for septicemia generally refers to a systemic disease associated with the presence of pathological microorganisms or toxins in the blood, which can include bacteria, viruses, or fungi.

  - Sepsis generally refers to SIRS due to infection.

  - Severe sepsis generally refers to sepsis with associated acute organ dysfunction.

- Determine whether the physician documented in the medical record the source of the infection, if known, and the organism, if identified.

- Review the medical record for documentation that indicates the presence of organ failure (e.g., acute renal failure, septic shock, acute respiratory or hepatic failure, metabolic encephalopathy related to sepsis) and code accordingly.

- Be sure to follow the sequencing guidelines for sepsis and SIRS as outlined in the official guidelines.

- Review the clinical information related to laboratory workup to see whether there are any positive blood cultures, which may be clinically significant or contaminants. Remember, absence of a positive blood culture does not preclude the diagnosis of sepsis being documented.

- Review for any predisposing factors (e.g., immunocompromised [as in diabetes], steroid therapy, malnutrition, immunoglobulin deficiency, chemotherapy), which should be clearly documented. If unclear, query the physician.

- Follow coding instructions if the physician documented any likelihood of a relationship to implanted devices, such as heart valve (endocarditis), indwelling Foley catheter, or vascular access device. Query the physician for clarification if there is conflicting or contrasting documentation. Do not assume that there is a complication by the mere fact that the patient has a urinary infection and an indwelling Foley catheter.

- Note that there is greater emphasis on sepsis within the health-care quality arena, and due to the risk of mortality, the early diagnosis of this condition can be key to improvements in patient outcomes. MedPAR data has shown an increase in the volume of sepsis admissions in the last several years; therefore, care should be taken to ensure accurate data is being captured, supported by clinical documentation and coding.

- Find codes for sepsis in Chapter 1, "Infectious and Parasitic Diseases (001–139)," in ICD-9-CM, Sixth Edition, valid from October 1, 2010, to September 30, 2011.

Stroke/Cerebrovascular Accident

- The word "stroke" has many synonyms, including brain attack, cerebral infarction, CVA, and even cerebral vascular disease. Because the language and wording is varied, it is important to review the medical record carefully, including the documentation of signs, symptoms, treatment, and prognosis.

- The medical condition of stroke occurs when the blood supply to the brain is stopped. The cause of this stoppage could be a blockage, a blood clot, or even a rupture of a vessel in the brain. A stroke is considered a medical emergency due to the potential for permanent damage that can occur, including, but not limited to, paralysis.

- In October 2004, changes occurred in the ICD-9-CM code indexing for the conditions of "stroke and CVA." The terms under ICD-9-CM code 436 were removed and reindexed to the default code of 434.91, cerebral artery occlusion, unspecified with cerebral infarction.

- Review the physician documentation carefully to determine whether the patient had a hemorrhagic stroke (e.g., intracerebral hemorrhage, subarachnoid hemorrhage) or had an occlusive or embolic cerebral infarction, as this will affect the code assignment and severity/acuity data.

- Review the medical record to determine whether there is a diagnosis of cerebral infarction, and whether it was due to primary intracerebral occlusion or carotid disease with embolism or cardioembolism.

- Check to see whether the patient had an evolving stroke that was aborted by enzyme or anticoagulant therapy; the ER record documentation may contain information relating to this situation.

- Look for documentation indicating that a study revealed carotid artery disease as the cause of the patient's current symptoms. Review this information closely for an indication that this hospitalization was because of current cerebral infarction or non-infarction cerebral embolism.

- Review the documentation carefully for indications of brain compression, which represents greater severity and ROM.

- Be aware of using the terms "reversible ischemic neurological deficit," "CVA," or simply "stroke," as they may be misconstrued and lead to codes that do not represent the true condition.

- Remember to assign ICD-9-CM codes for the residuals from an old CVA as additional codes for a patient admitted with a current CVA. Instructions allow the coding of residuals from an acute CVA even when present in the current admission and is resolved by the time the patient is discharged.

- Assign procedure code 99.10, injection or infusion of thrombo-lytic agent, if tissue plasminogen activator is given/infused or injected.

- Look for codes for cerebral vascular accident/infarction or stroke in Chapter 6, "Diseases of Nervous System and Sense Organs (320–389)," in ICD-9-CM, Sixth Edition, valid from October 1, 2010, to September 30, 2011.

Symptoms

- Remember that ICD-9-CM codes for symptoms, signs, and ill-defined conditions are from Chapter 16 of ICD-9-CM, Sixth Edition, and cannot be used as principal diagnoses or reasons for outpatient encounters when the related diagnoses have been established. Understanding this coding convention can ensure coding accuracy.

- One of the core competencies of a coding professional is to understand disease processes, which includes understanding the signs and symptoms. This will help in knowing when and when not to assign a symptom code that would otherwise be integral to a disease.

- Look for documentation that distinctly identifies the relationship between signs and symptoms on admission and the diagnoses determined after workup.

- Follow coding guidelines for correct sequencing if, after reviewing the documentation, you believe a symptom may be due to either of two (or more) diagnoses. If necessary, query the physician.

- Obtain clarification from the physician if the documentation indicates that a patient's symptoms could be due to several diseases, none of which meets the definition of a principal diagnosis.

- Determine whether the physician documented the diagnosis that he or she believed existed whenever studies or treatments were ordered while the patient was in the hospital.

- Review the medical record for documentation of cardiac or cardiorespiratory arrest that identifies the most likely cause of the event. If the cause is indeterminate, query the physician for what he or she believed to be the origin of the arrest (e.g., the central nervous system).

Syncope

- Clarify with the physician whether the patient had an identifiable event, such as post-micturition syncope, cough-related syncope, a frightening event, or sudden positional change. If the patient did, query the physician to document that information in the medical record as the cause of the syncope.

- Review the documentation carefully to help determine whether dehydration was the cause of syncope, as this is a common problem in the elderly. In addition, review the medical record documentation for an indication of an arrhythmia or drug-drug interaction, as this is also common in the elderly. In the case of an arrhythmia, query the physician for the cause if known.

- Review the ER documentation and admitting H&P when syncope has occurred to help determine whether the patient had a trip or fall. In addition, look for information about choking. If this information exists in the ER documentation or admitting H&P, ask the physician to document it in the medical record.

- Review the documentation and look for indication of an acute MI, stroke, or sepsis. If one of these conditions is documented, query the physician to find out whether that was the cause of the episode.

- Code syncope without any further clarification to ICD-9-CM code 780.2, syncope and collapse.

Trauma

- Be aware that trauma coding often involves detailed review of ER and inpatient record documentation. Patients may have multiple traumatic injuries that need medical attention and the assignment of multiple ICD-9-CM codes. There may also be multiple consultations in the medical record from a variety of specialists.

- Review the emergency trauma record carefully.

- Review the documentation for information about a concussion or a transient loss of consciousness/the specific length of time during which consciousness was lost. Nursing notes may provide some clues, although you cannot code directly from the nursing notes; coders may need to query the physician for clarification.

- Code all rib fractures. Note that, in trauma cases, multiple fractures may have occurred.

- Read over the patient vitals. If hypovolemic shock occurred, query the physician for additional documentation or clarification if necessary.

- Review carefully the documentation when coding an acute respiratory failure in a trauma case to determine whether the respiratory failure is due to the trauma or the drugs, and follow the ICD-9-CM guidelines.

Summary

The work around clinical documentation and coding accuracy involves dedicated staff who will collaborate and communicate together. With the growing compliance and regulatory audits, the healthcare industry and providers need to be more diligent with regard to the language used in clinical documentation and the resulting code(s). The electronic health record, coupled with documentation improvement efforts and computer-assisted coding, will help provide some new solutions to these challenges. The use of natural language process (NLP) technology, even with the electronic health record, can offer some solutions and opportunities worth exploring. With ICD-10 implementation coming soon, this is the time to initiate a dialog and energize new efforts that can impact and/or improve the overall documentation and coded data. Whichever means and methods you use, it's important to have regular and frequent communication with providers. Being dedicated and persistent in this area will produce results, not only at your institution or within your practice, but for healthcare in general.

Endnote

The Cooperating Parties (AHIMA, AHA, CMS, and the National Center for Health Statistics) publish official guidelines in *Coding Clinic for ICD-9-CM,* available from the AHA. These guidelines are also available in the ICD-9-CM CD-ROM offered by the U.S. Government Printing Office.

General References

American Hospital Association. *AHA Coding Clinic for ICD-9-CM, 1987–2011.* Chicago, IL: American Hospital Association.

Brown, F. (2011). *ICD-9-CM Coding Handbook With Answers.* Chicago, IL: American Hospital Association.

Centers for Disease Control and Prevention. *The International Classification of Diseases, 9th Revision, Clinical Modification.* Atlanta, GA: The Centers for Disease Control and Prevention.

Gold, R.S. (2005). *Documentation Strategies to Support Severity of Illness: Ensure an Accurate Professional Profile.* Marblehead, MA: HCPro, Inc.

U.S. Department of Health and Human Services. (October 2010). *ICD-9-CM Official Guidelines for Coding and Reporting, Effective October 2010.* Washington, DC: U.S. Department of Health and Human Services.

ADDITIONAL RESOURCES

Certified Coding Specialist (CCS): Coding Core Competencies

The following is a list of the coding competency domains as identified by AHIMA:

- **DOMAIN I.** Health Information Documentation

- **DOMAIN II.** Diagnosis Coding

- **DOMAIN III.** Procedure Coding

- **DOMAIN IV.** Regulatory Guidelines and Reporting Requirements for Acute Care (Inpatient) Service

- **DOMAIN V.** Regulatory Guidelines and Reporting Requirements for Outpatient Services

- **DOMAIN VI.** Data Quality and Management

- **DOMAIN VII.** Information and Communication Technologies

- **DOMAIN VIII.** Privacy, Confidentiality, Legal, and Ethical Issues

- **DOMAIN IX.** Compliance

Coding Tip Sheet: New FY11 BMI V Codes

- **V85.41** – Body Mass Index 40.0–44.9, adult

- **V85.42** – Body Mass Index 45.0–49.9, adult

- **V85.43** – Body Mass Index 50.0–59.9, adult

- **V85.44** – Body Mass Index 60.0–69.9, adult

- **V85.45** – Body Mass Index 70 and over, adult

Notes:

- It is important to capture documentation of patient BMI

- BMI can be assigned based on documentation from nonphysician providers (refer to the *Official Coding Guidelines*)

- An associated clinical diagnosis/condition is also needed when reporting or coding BMI

Sample Physician Query

Coding clarification form: Pathology diagnosis

Please respond within 48 hours from *** (date of query)

Medical record number:

Hospital account record:

Patient name:

Admit date:

Discharge date:

To: **From:**

Department: **HIM department ext.:**

Clarification of medical record documentation is required to meet compliance, to ensure accuracy of coding, and to reflect the severity of illness and risk of mortality of your patient.

We received a pathology report that indicated potentially significant clinical findings. The pathology report may not have been available for review prior to the patient's discharge. Please review the pathology report and document whether there is any clinical significance to the pathology findings.

For hospital inpatient coding, we are not allowed to code from pathology or laboratory reports. It is acceptable for the physician to establish a hospital diagnosis from pathology results returned after discharge based on specimens collected during the hospital stay.

Please document your response below:

Physician's signature: _____ **Date:** _____

Thank you.

NOTES

NOTES